THE ALLERGIC PRINCE

A Customizable Tale of Food Allergies

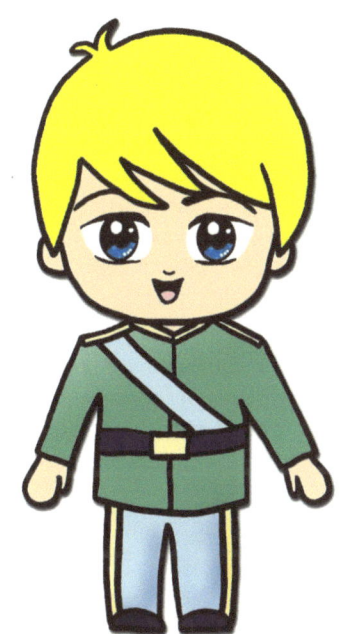

Written and Illustrated by

Jennifer Chung and Keira Chung

www.AllergicPrince.com

Available from Amazon.com and other online stores.

Summary: When Prince Ethan is tempted by multiple situations involving food, he learns to summon the willpower within to keep himself safe from allergic foods.

For:

Raymond & Barbara who taught us we could achieve anything

and

The staff at Sean N. Parker Center for Allergy and Asthma Research
at Stanford University
for giving us the world.

How to customize this book:
To create a story to which your child can fully relate, fill in your child's allergic foods, symptoms, and safe snacks into the blank spaces (ballpoint pens work best) on pages 14, 16, and 31.

Examples of allergic foods: milk, peanuts, almonds, eggs, soy, wheat, sesame seeds, fish, shellfish, etc.
Examples of allergic symptoms: itchy mouth, hives, vomiting, stomachache, wheezing, trouble breathing, etc.
Examples of safe snacks: fruits, carrots, crackers, yogurt, etc.

This book belongs to:

_____

"Hooray! The day I've been waiting for is finally here!" yelled Prince Ethan as he climbed into the royal carriage.

Ethan's mommy had summoned the carriage to bring him to Prince Jordan's birthday party.

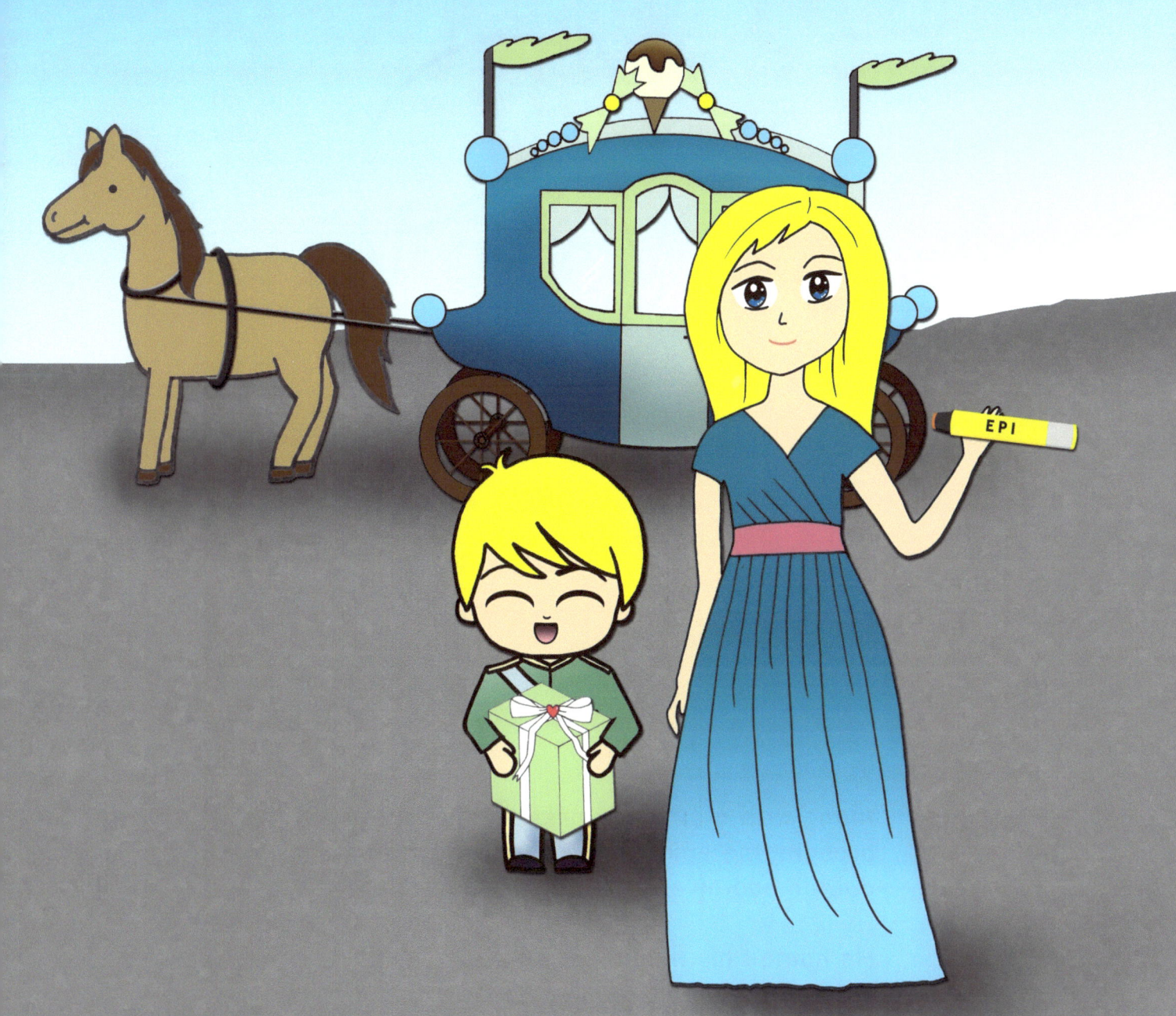

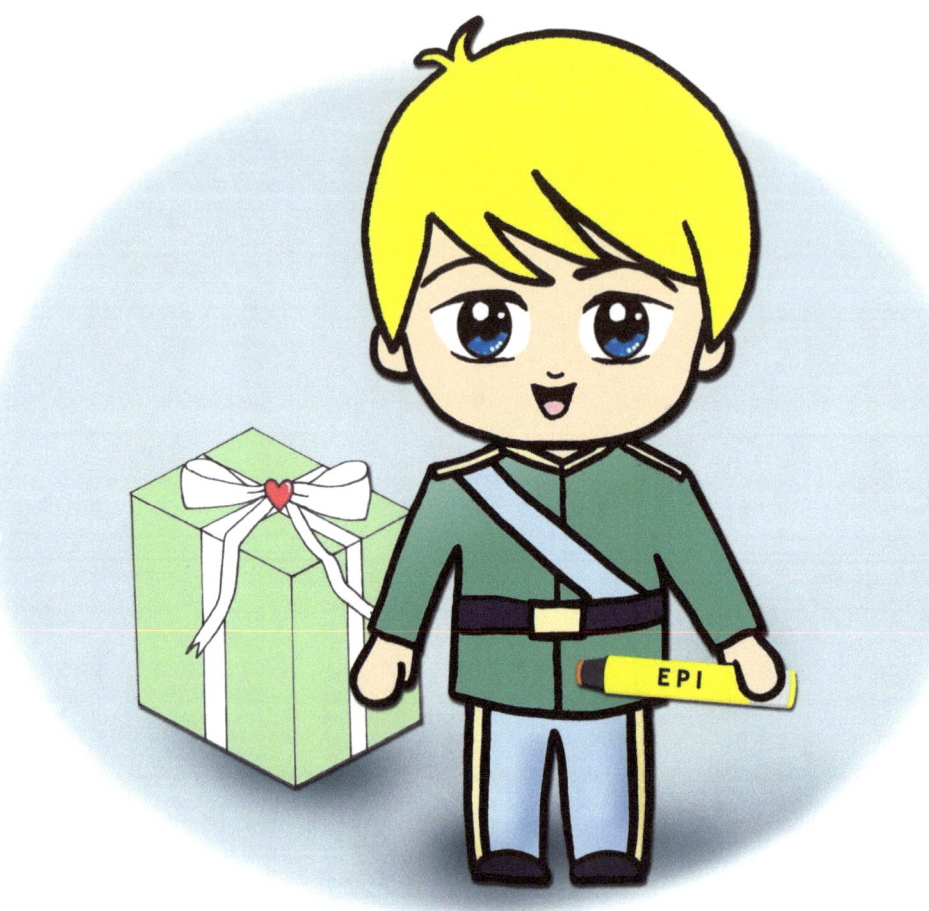

Along with a birthday present, Ethan also brought the epinephrine medicine that his doctor had given him for his food allergies.

He named his medicine, *Epi*. Epi was his emergency medicine in case he accidentally ate food that he was allergic to.

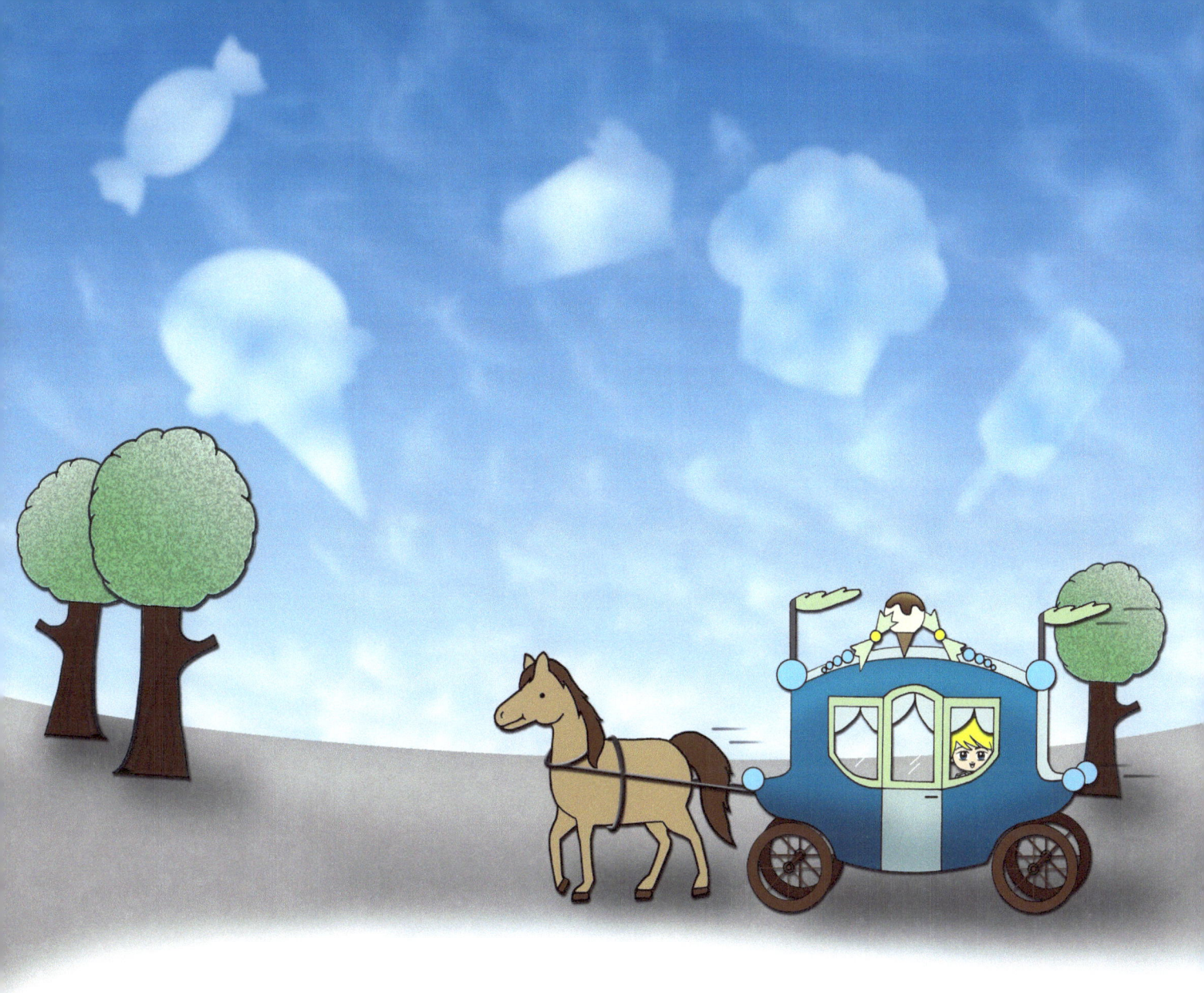

Looking out the window of the carriage,
Ethan watched as cloud shapes passed by.

It felt like the longest ride ever, until Ethan finally spotted Jordan's castle. As he passed through the castle gate, his heart raced faster. What will the party be like? He wondered. Will I be allergic to the cake?

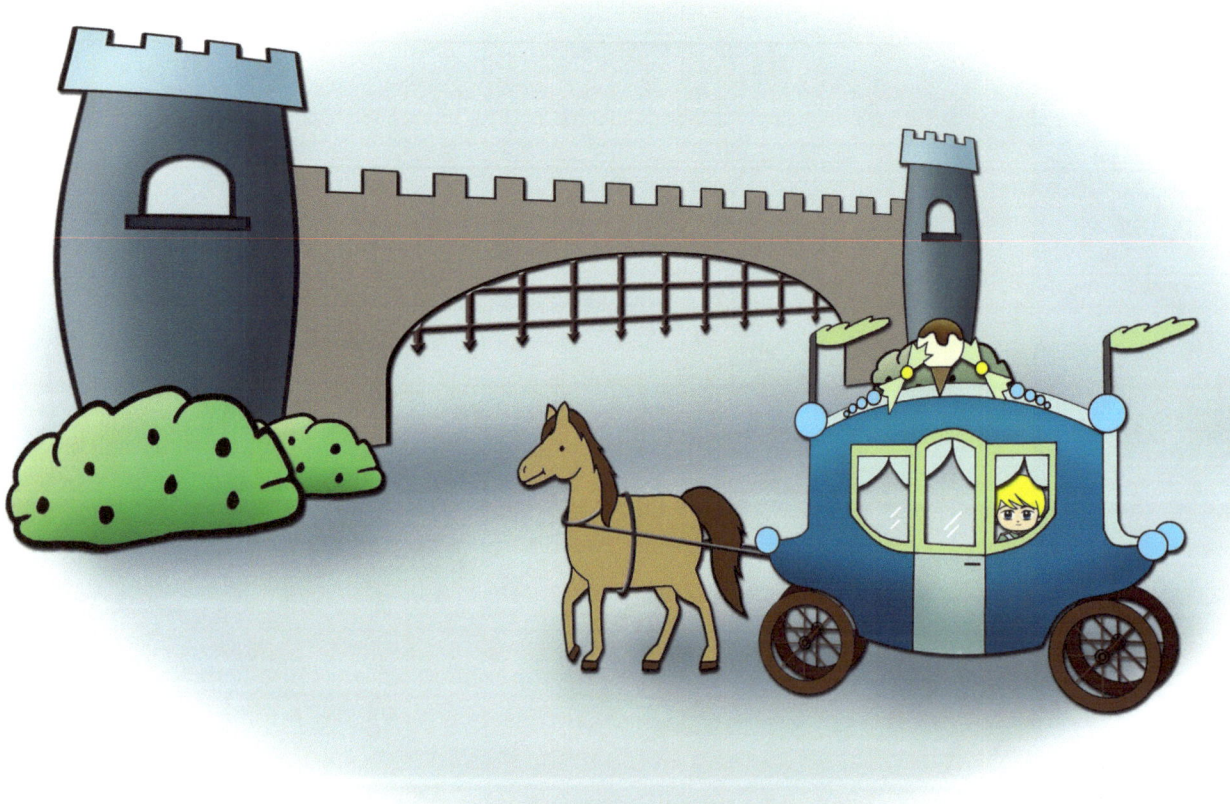

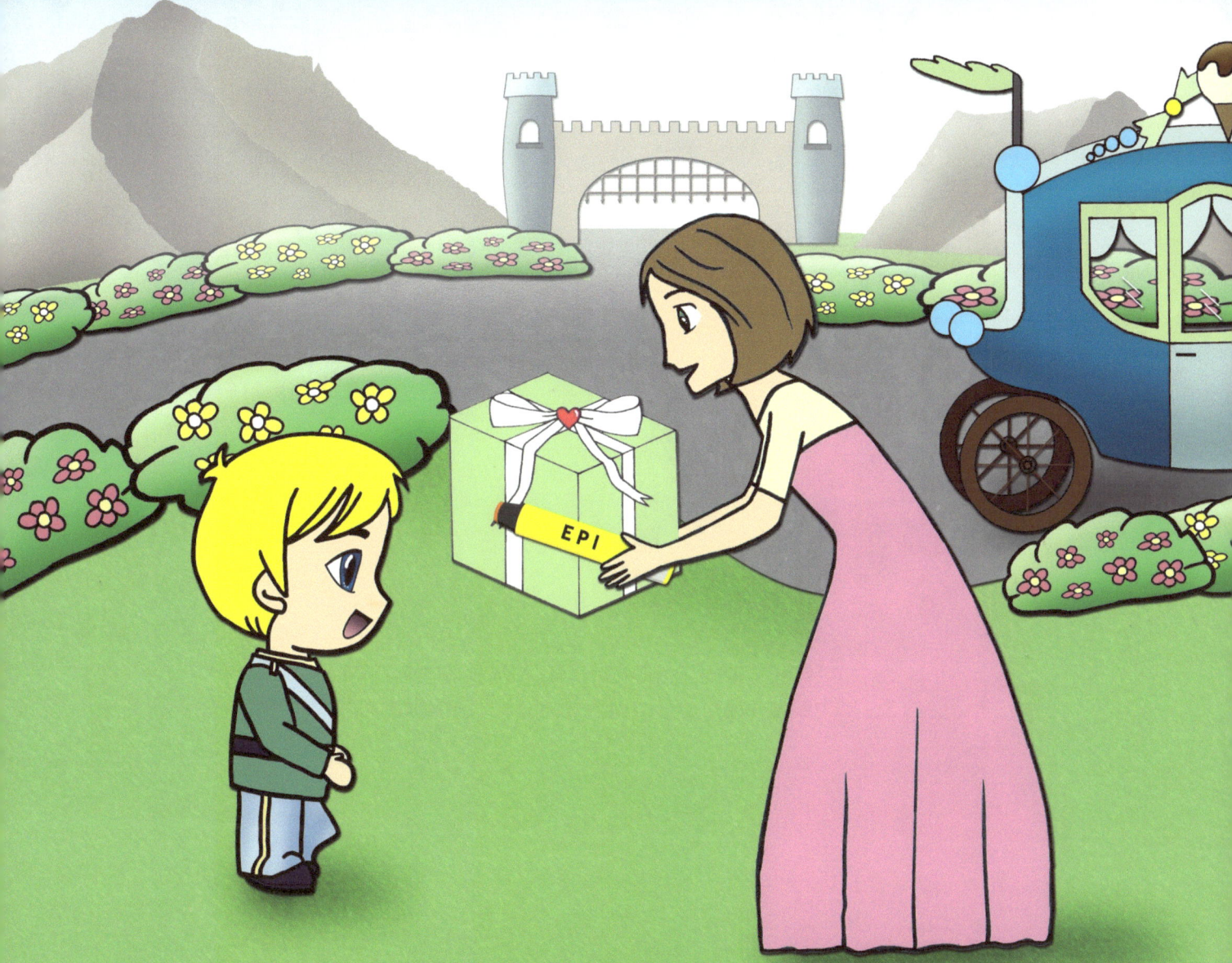

At last, the carriage came to a stop and Ethan
excitedly hopped off. He handed both Epi and
the birthday present to Jordan's mommy, who
came to welcome him into their castle grounds.

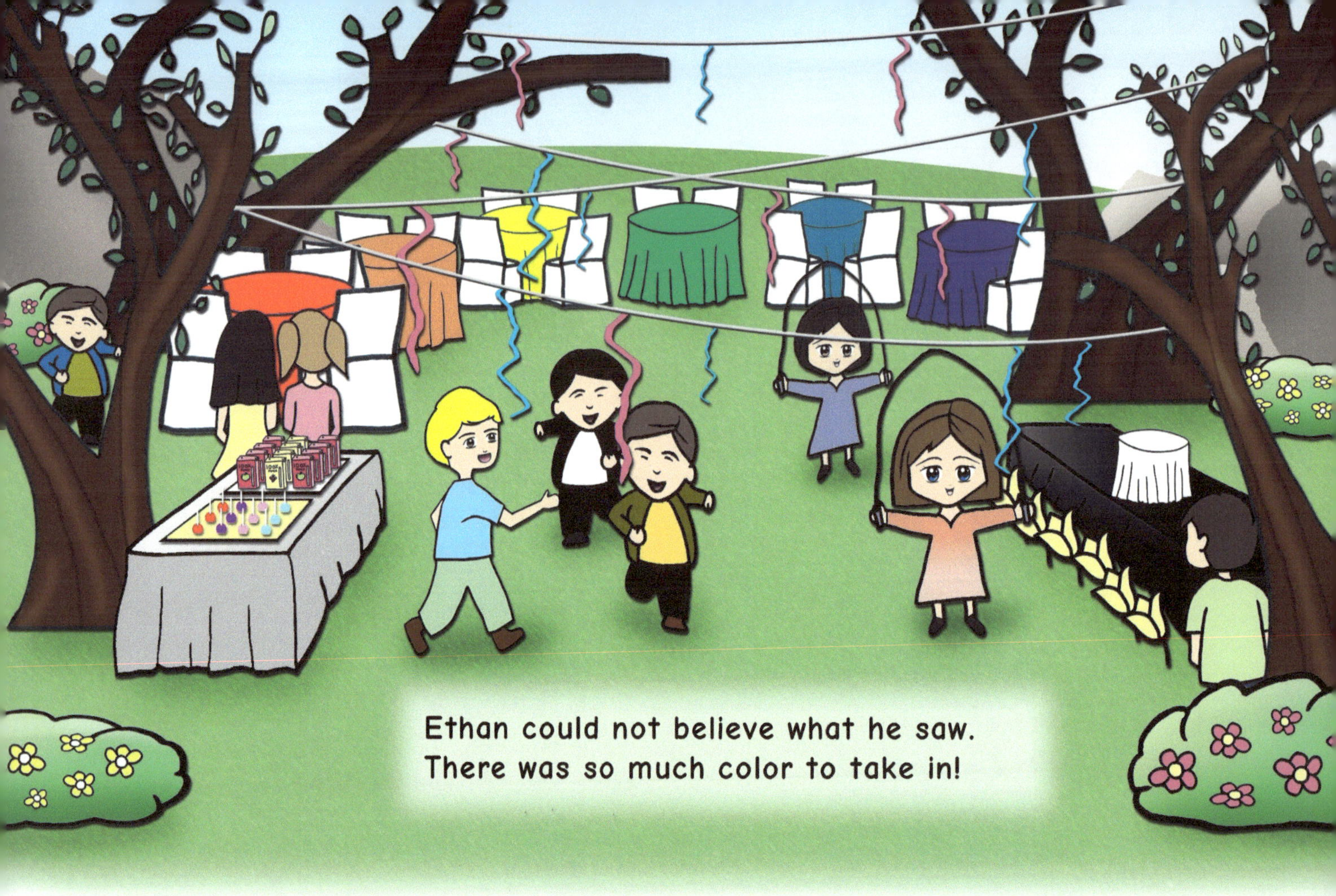

Ethan could not believe what he saw.
There was so much color to take in!

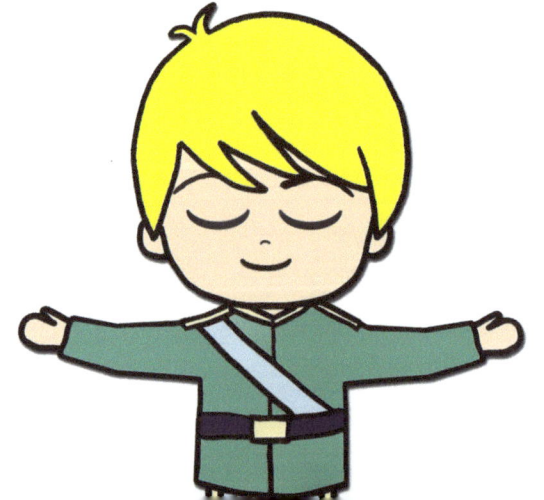

To savor the moment, he closed
his eyes and took a deep breath.

The feeling of fresh air and the
sound of children's laughter
surrounded him.

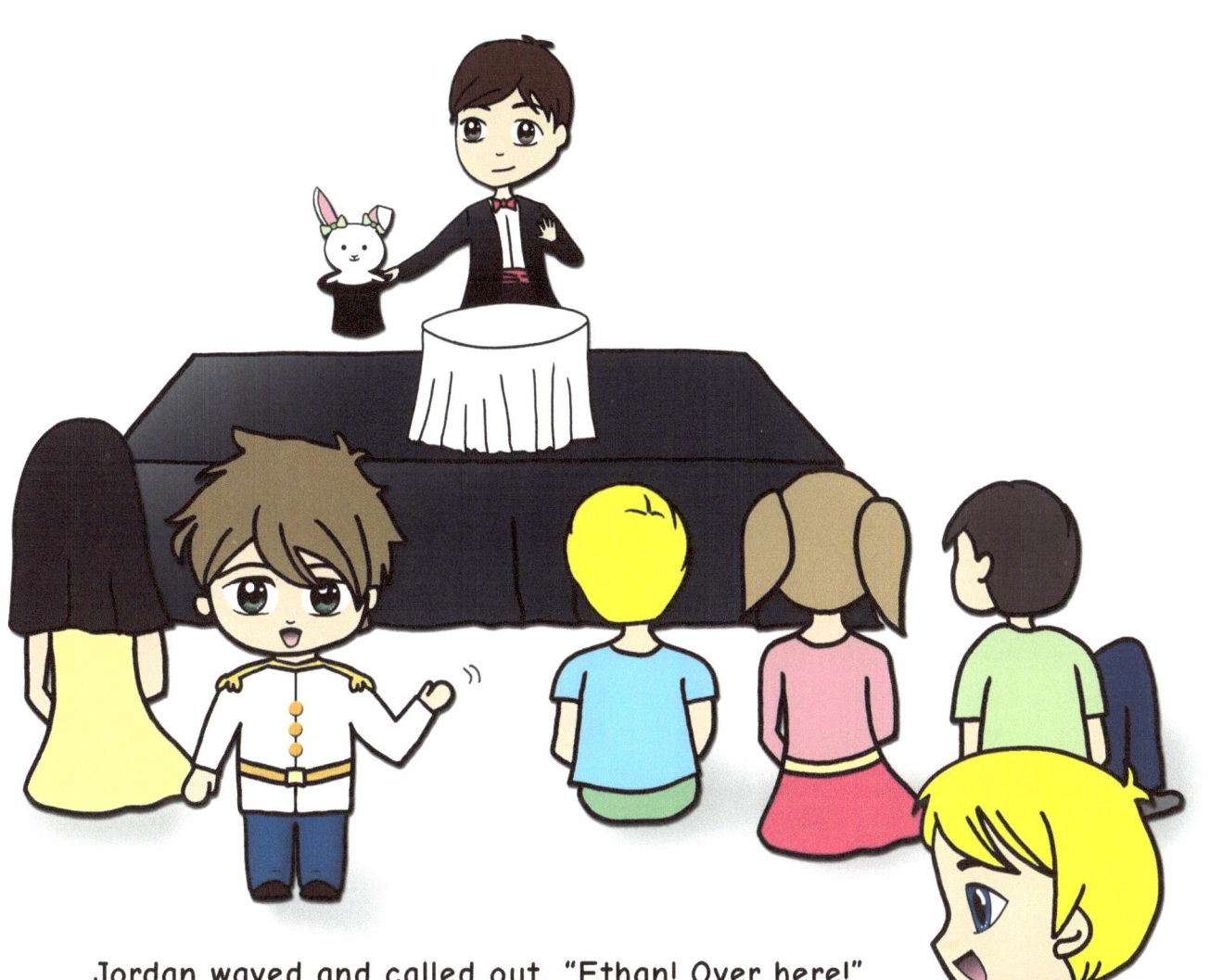

Jordan waved and called out, "Ethan! Over here!"

Ethan looked around, then ran over to Jordan
and sat next to him to watch the magic show.

As the magician pulled a white bunny out of a hat,
the children oohed and aahed in amazement.

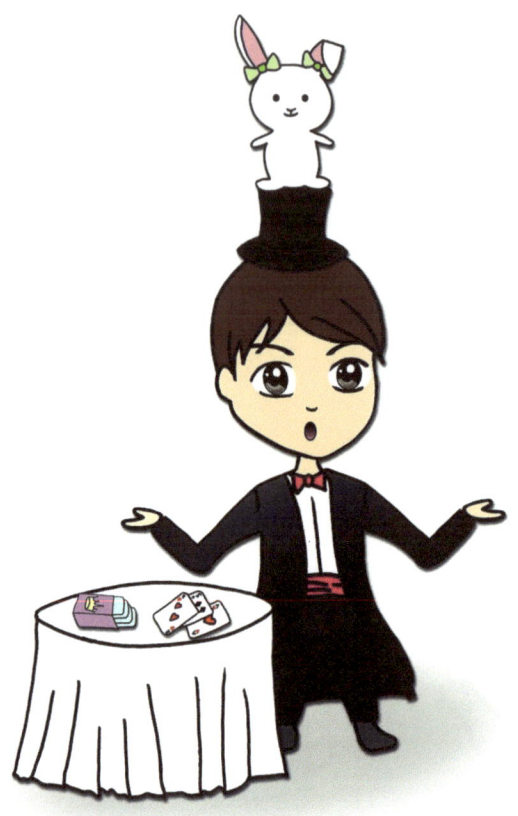

To prepare for his next trick, the magician placed the bunny on the table and went to find his deck of cards. Without warning, the bunny hopped away.

The magician looked around and asked the children, "Do you know where my bunny went?"

All at once, the children started laughing.

After the fun-filled magic show, it was time for the birthday cake. Ethan screamed as he jumped up and down, clapping his hands. Three magnificent layers of chocolate cake decorated with blue, gold, and white frosting stood before him.

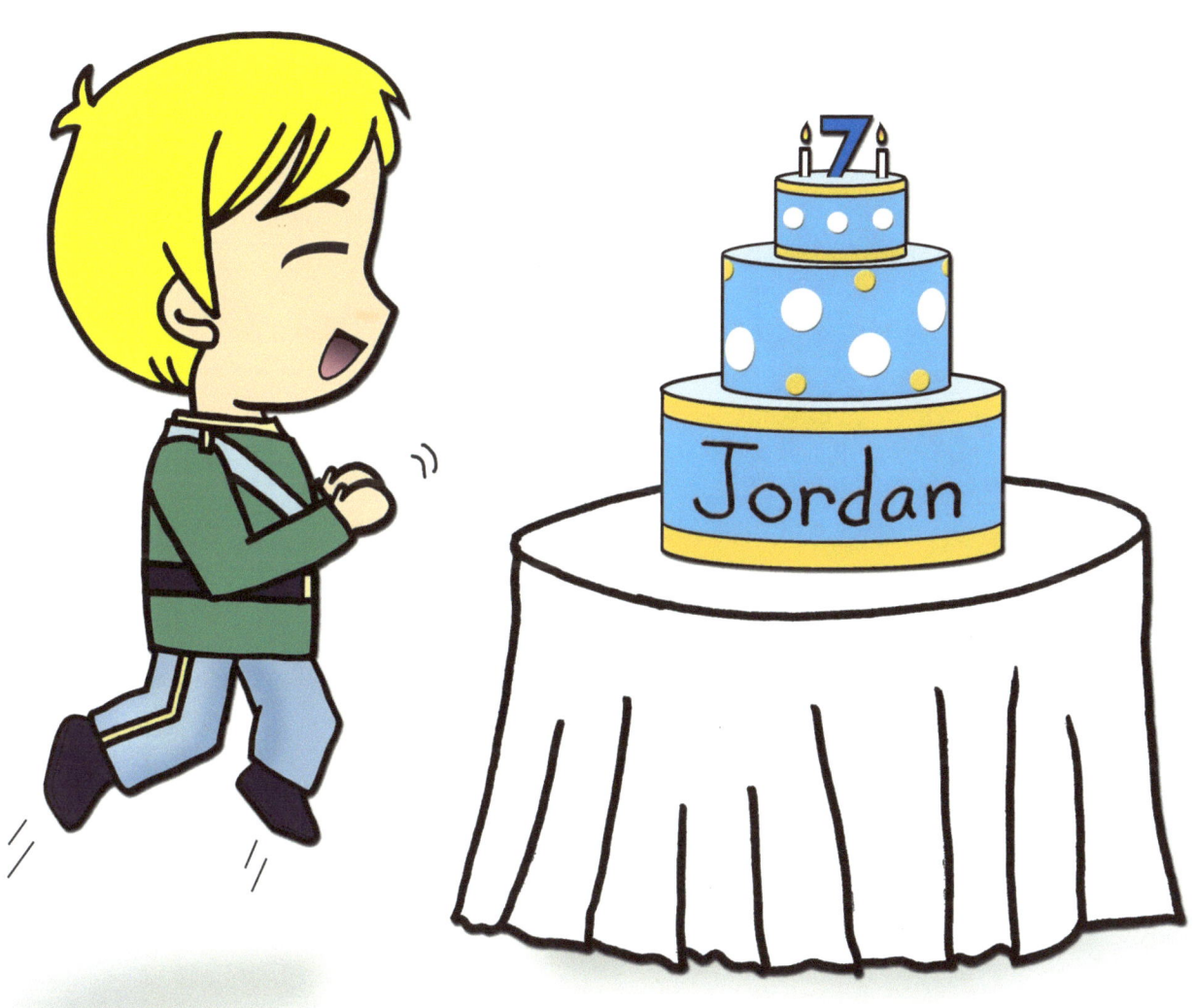

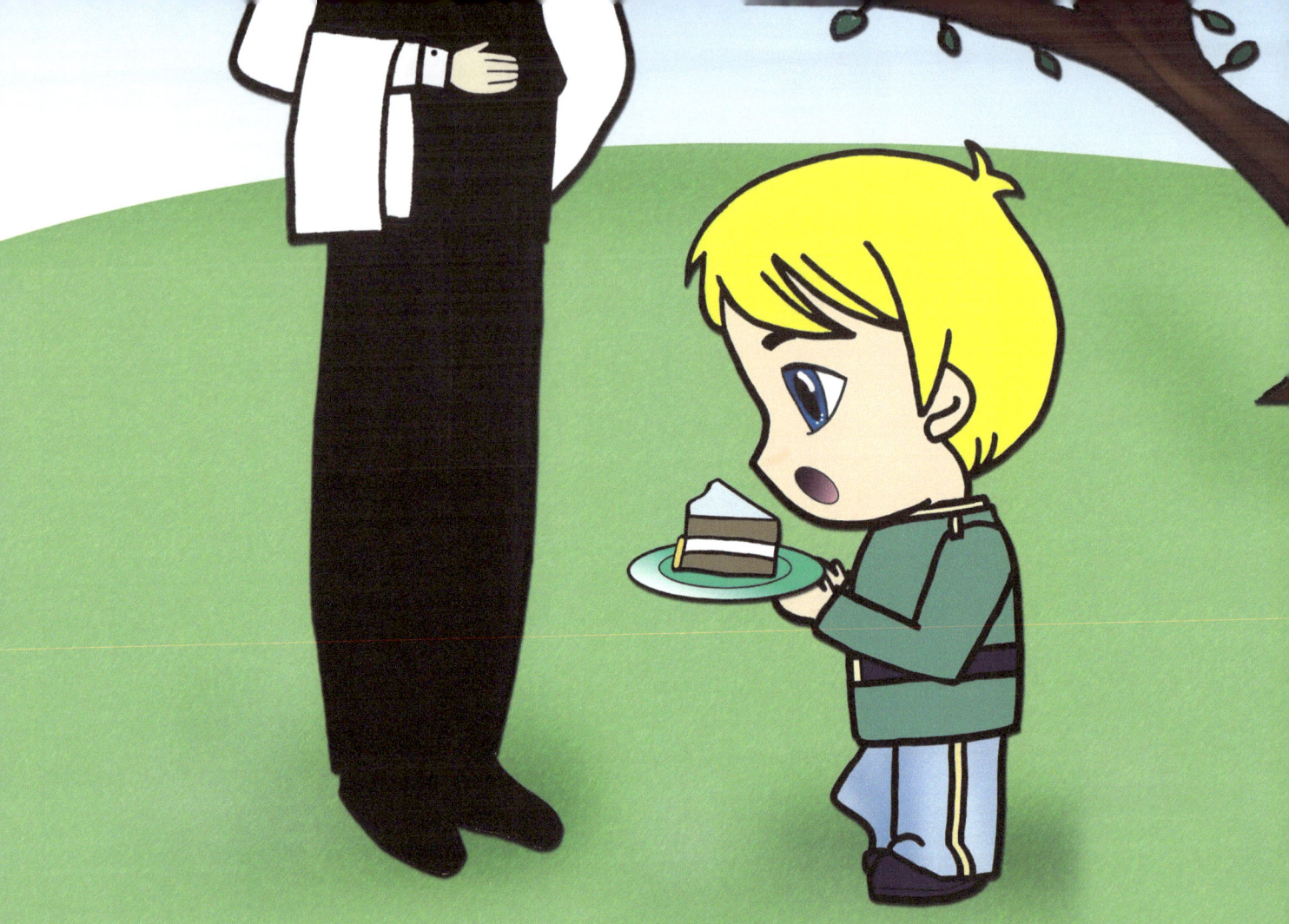

Ethan stared with huge eyes at the piece of cake that was handed to him. What should I do? What *can* I do? He remembered his food allergies, but the cake looked both delicious and so harmless.

He did not see any _____
in the cake.   [fill in allergic foods here]

Standing alone, Ethan glanced around as he held the slice of cake. He took a chance and scooped the biggest bite ever and placed it in his mouth. It was scrumptious!

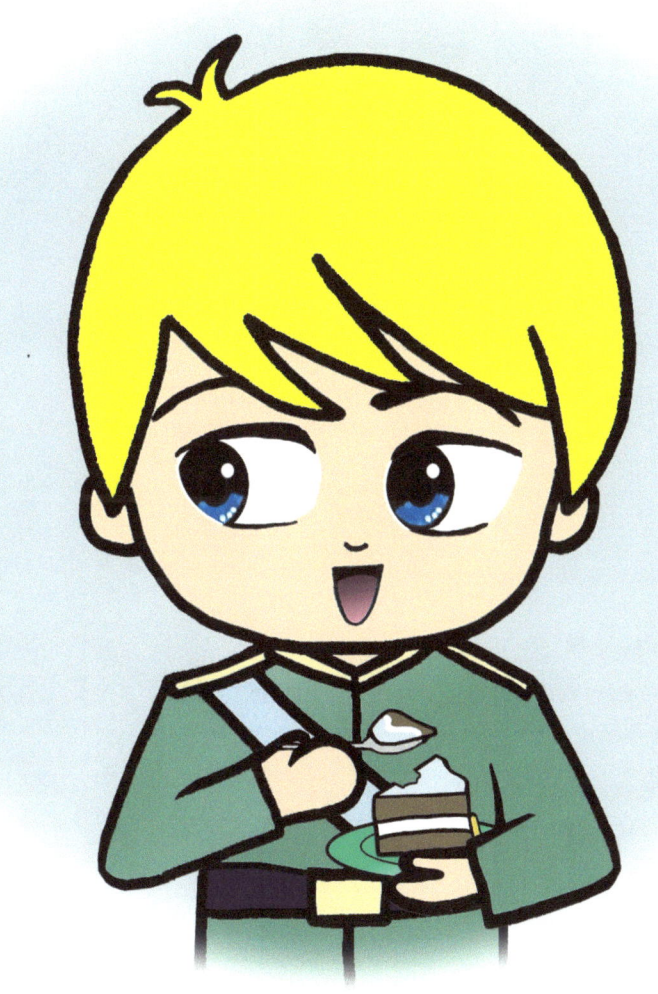

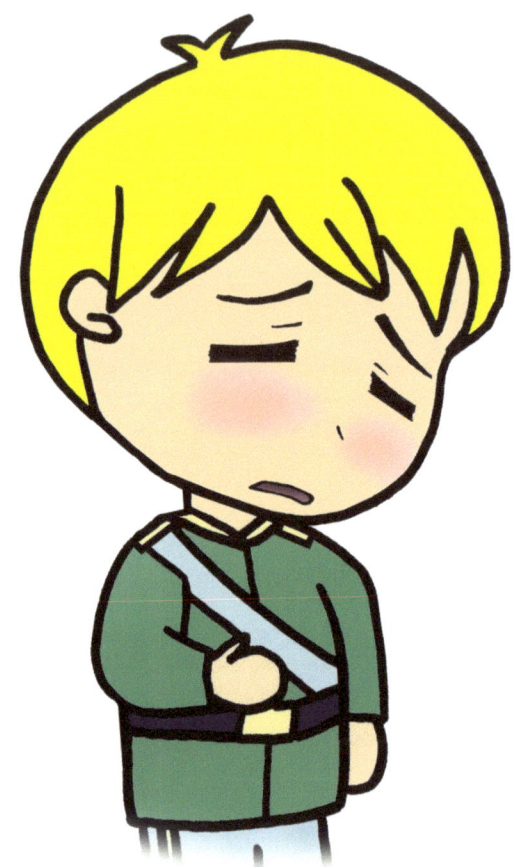

In an instant, everything changed. Ethan felt sick and realized that he was having an allergic reaction.

He recognized the symptoms of _____.
He needed help!

[fill in allergic symptoms here]

Ethan ran to the butler and told him,
"I'm having an allergic reaction... and I
need my Epi!"

He notified Jordan's mommy immediately.

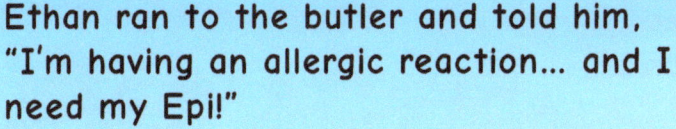

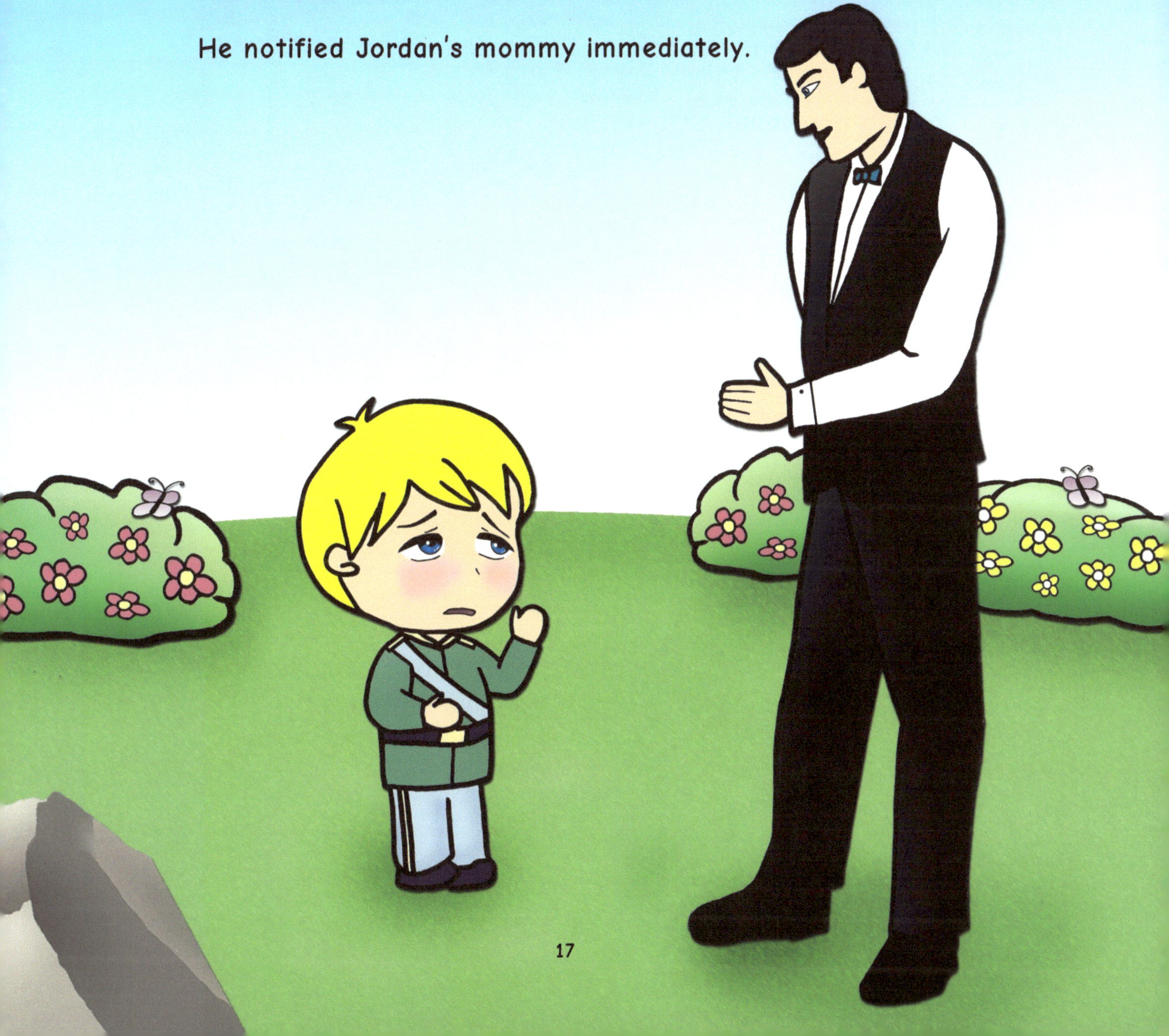

17

Jordan's mommy rushed over and injected Ethan's Epi into his leg.

Jordan came over to see what all the commotion was about and saw that his friend was in trouble. He wanted to stay with Ethan, but realized he had to do a very important job first.

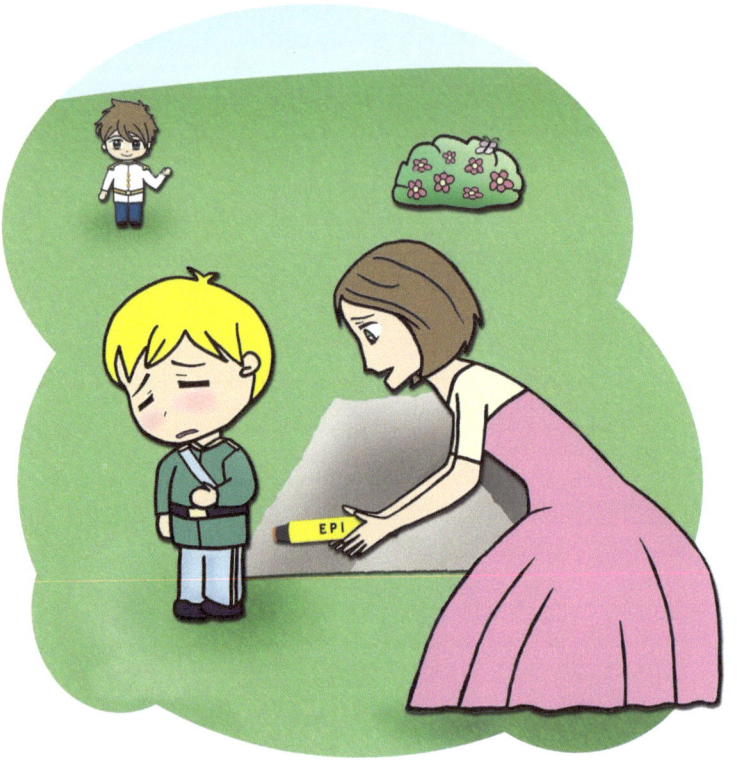

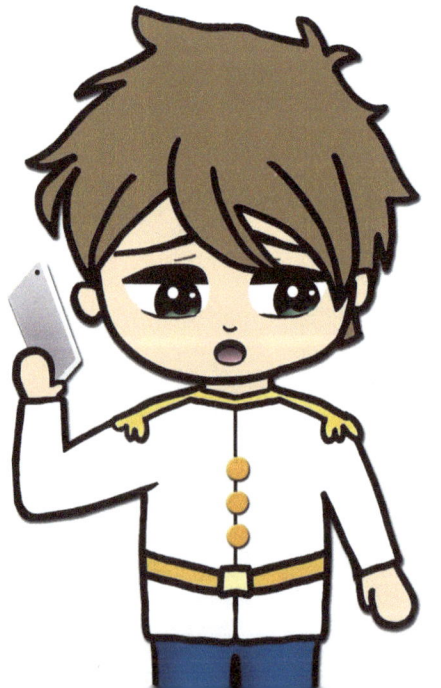

He went to the phone and called Ethan's mommy to tell her what had happened.

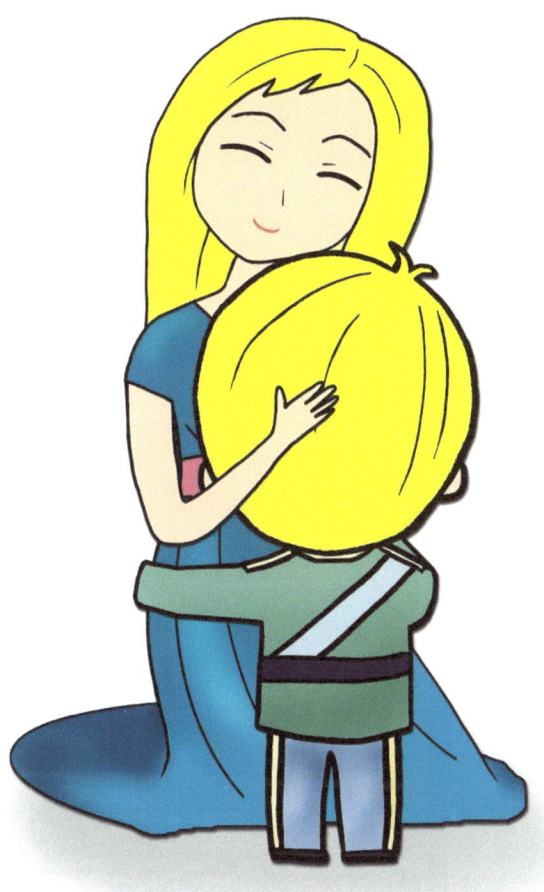

Although he was still scared, Ethan began to feel better. When his mommy finally arrived to bring him to the Royal Hospital, Ethan sank into her arms.

"I'm so glad you're here," whispered Ethan.

That night, after the hospital visit, Ethan was glad to go home so that he could cuddle with his favorite teddy bear. He ate a quick dinner and went to bed early to have a good night of sleep.

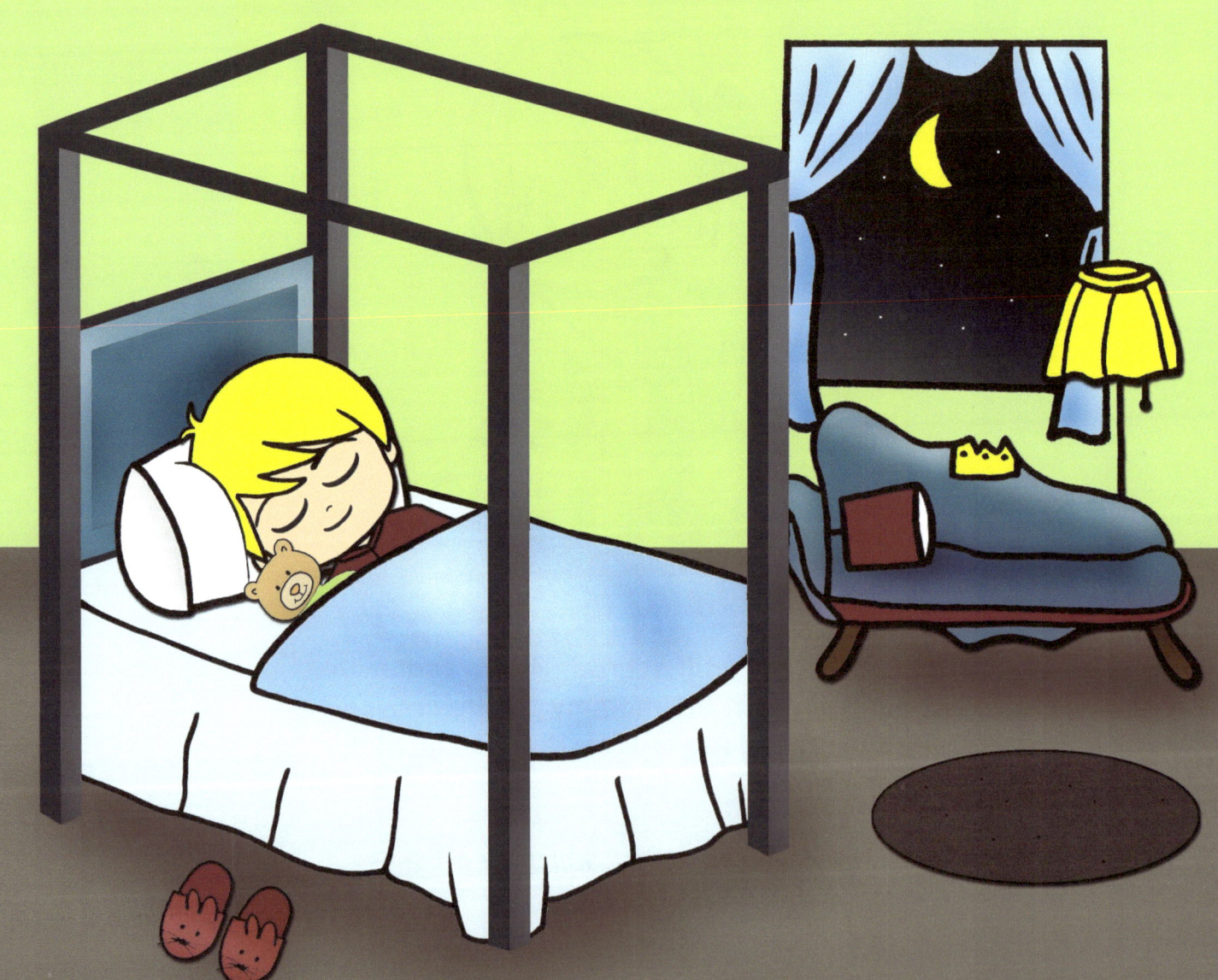

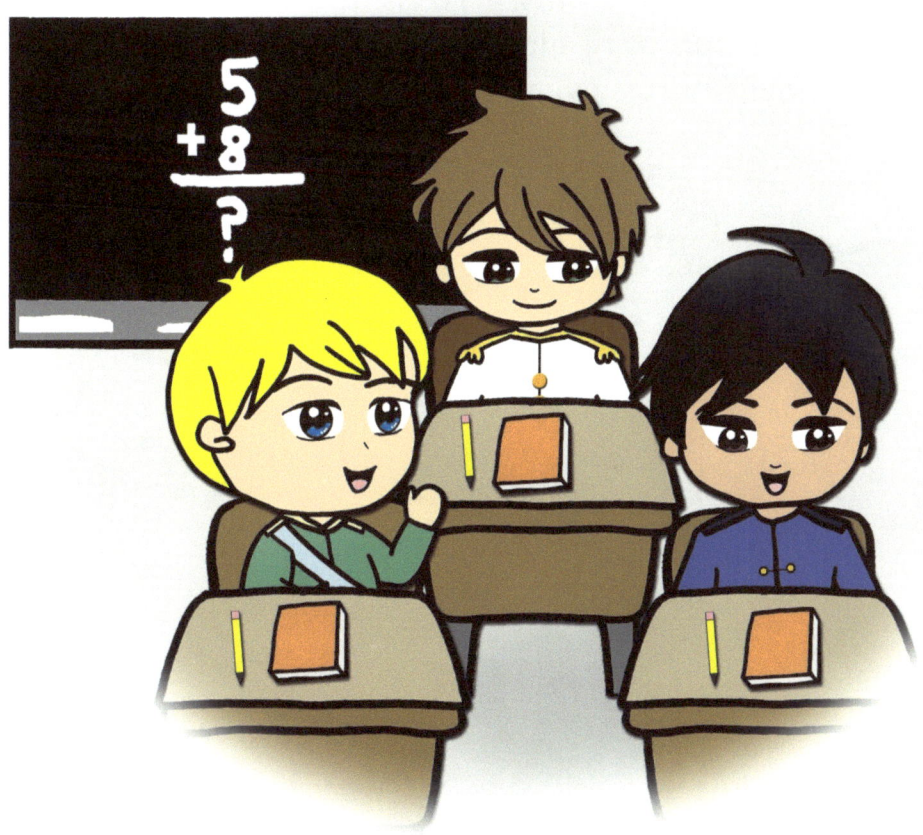

The next morning, Ethan woke up feeling refreshed. He got dressed and ate breakfast, then hopped onto the carriage, ready for a new day at school. When he reached Royal Academy School, he noticed a new boy he had never seen before. His name was Prince Kyle.

"Kyle, want to come to my castle for a play date tomorrow?" asked Ethan. "Jordan will be there too."

"That would be excellent, I will ask my mother," replied Kyle.

When Kyle and his mommy arrived at Ethan's castle,
Ethan and Jordan were already playing with a soccer
ball. They quickly ran over to greet Kyle.

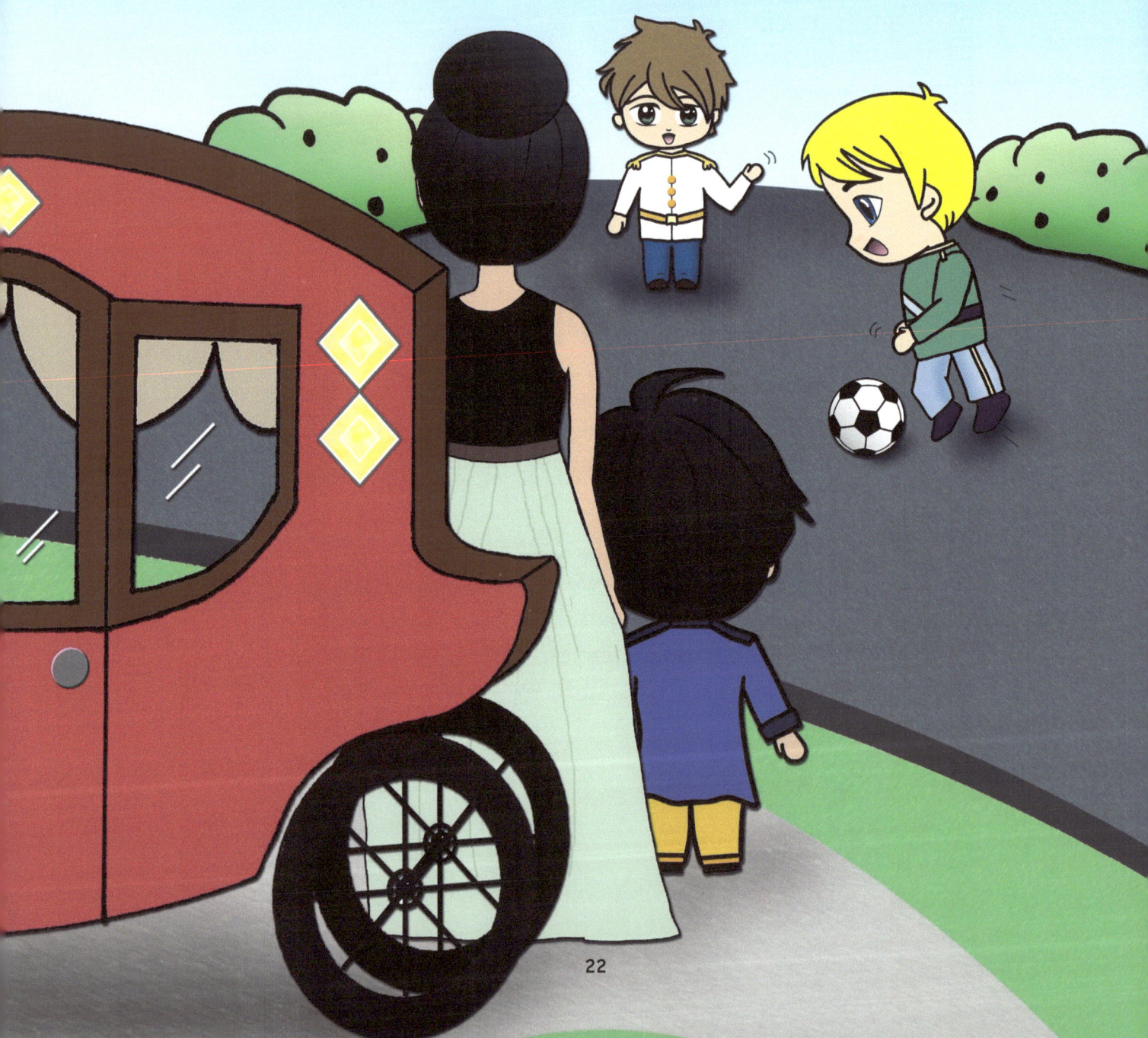

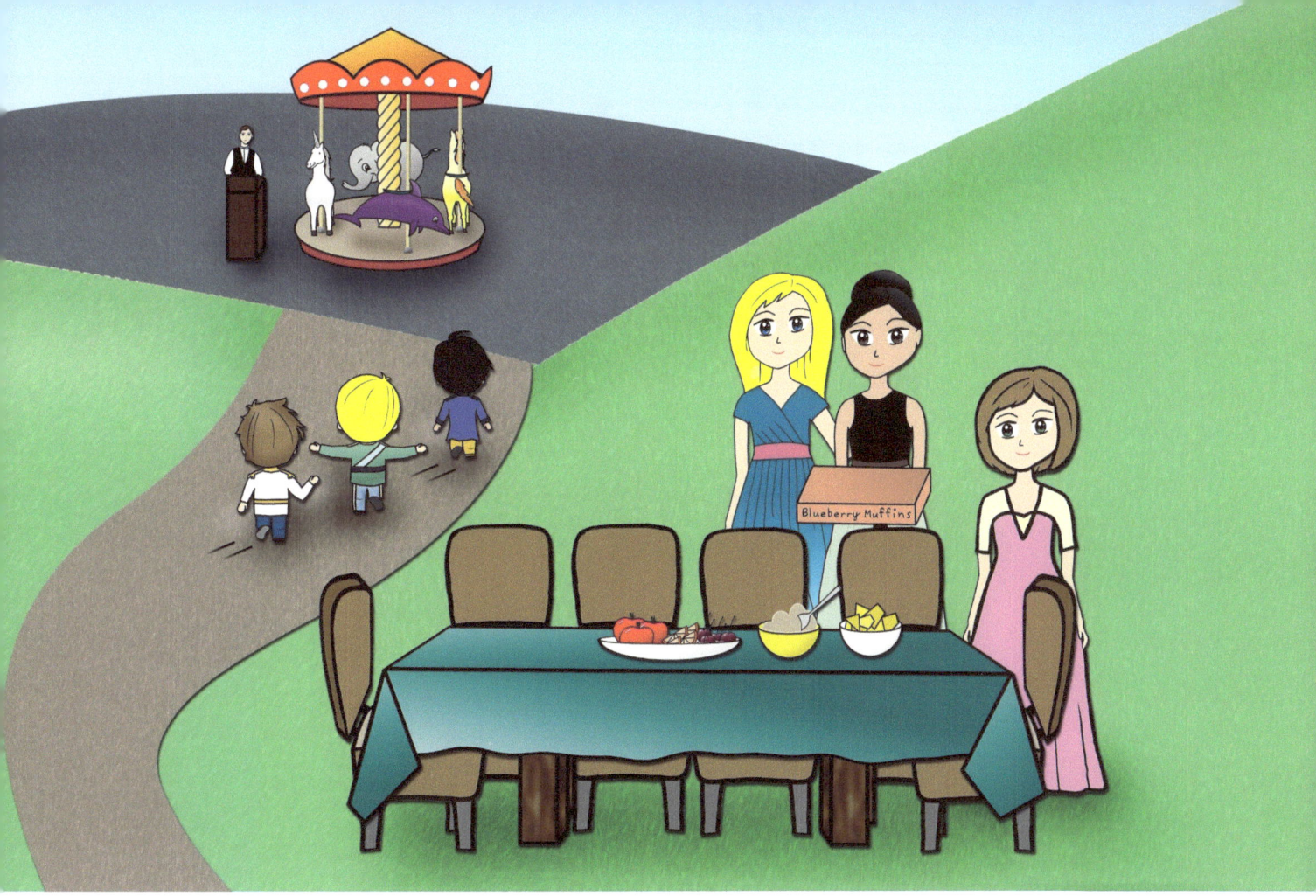

The three boys raced to the carousel while the three mommies sat down for a nice long chat.

"I would like the yellow horse," stated Kyle.

"Purple dolphin, you're mine!" cried Ethan.

"The white unicorn for me!" shouted Jordan.

The music began and off the boys went! The carousel spun faster and faster, around and around, again and again.

"Woohoo! This is the best!" cried Jordan.

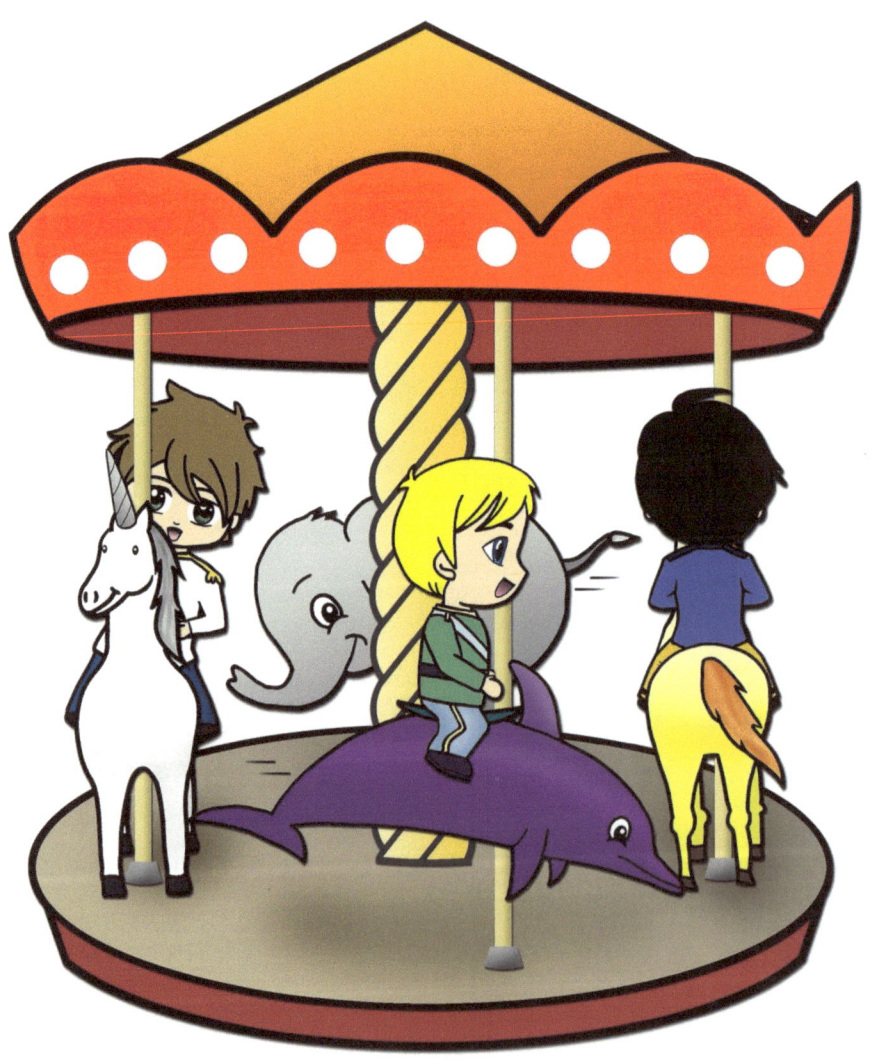

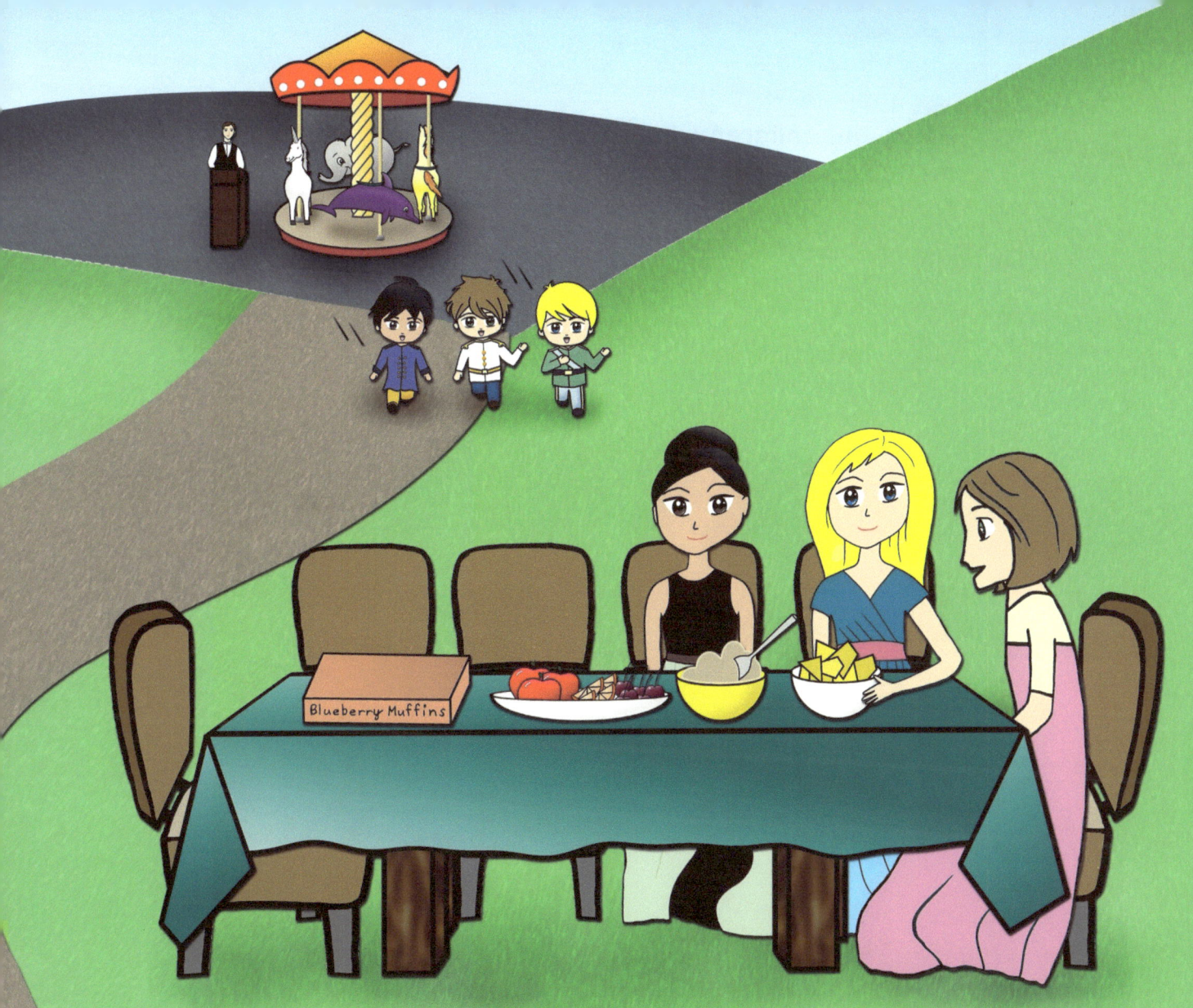

After a few more times around the carousel, the boys got off, looked at each other, and declared in unison, "We're starving!" They headed towards their mommies sitting at the picnic table.

After the children wiped their hands clean, Kyle's mommy took out a box of muffins that she bought from the bakery.

"Who would like a muffin?" she asked.

"Ooh! May I have one?" asked Kyle.

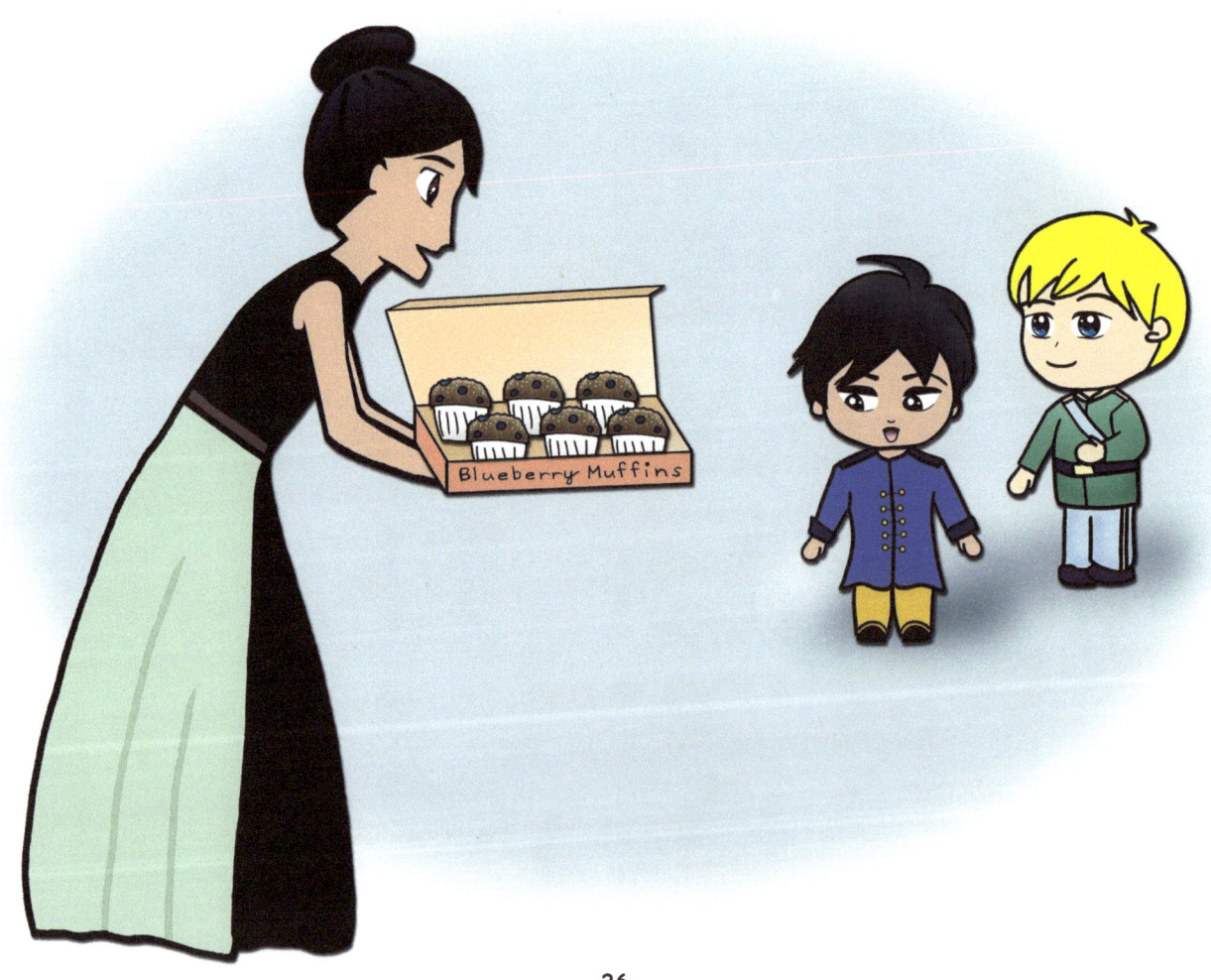

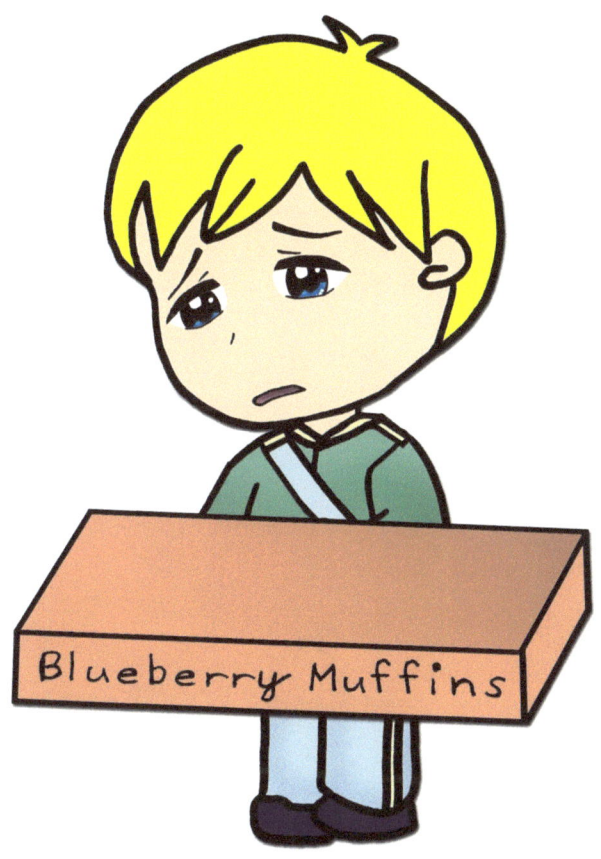

Ethan looked all over the box, but he did not see a list of ingredients. He could almost taste the blueberries and sugar crunch topping, yet he remembered his food allergies. An allergic reaction was definitely not something he wanted to go through again. He lowered his head and gazed at the ground.

"No, thank you," he replied softly.

Confused, Kyle's mommy asked him why.

Ethan hesitated, unsure of what to say, then muttered, "Well... I really want to try a muffin, but I have food allergies... and I have to be extra careful when ingredients aren't listed."

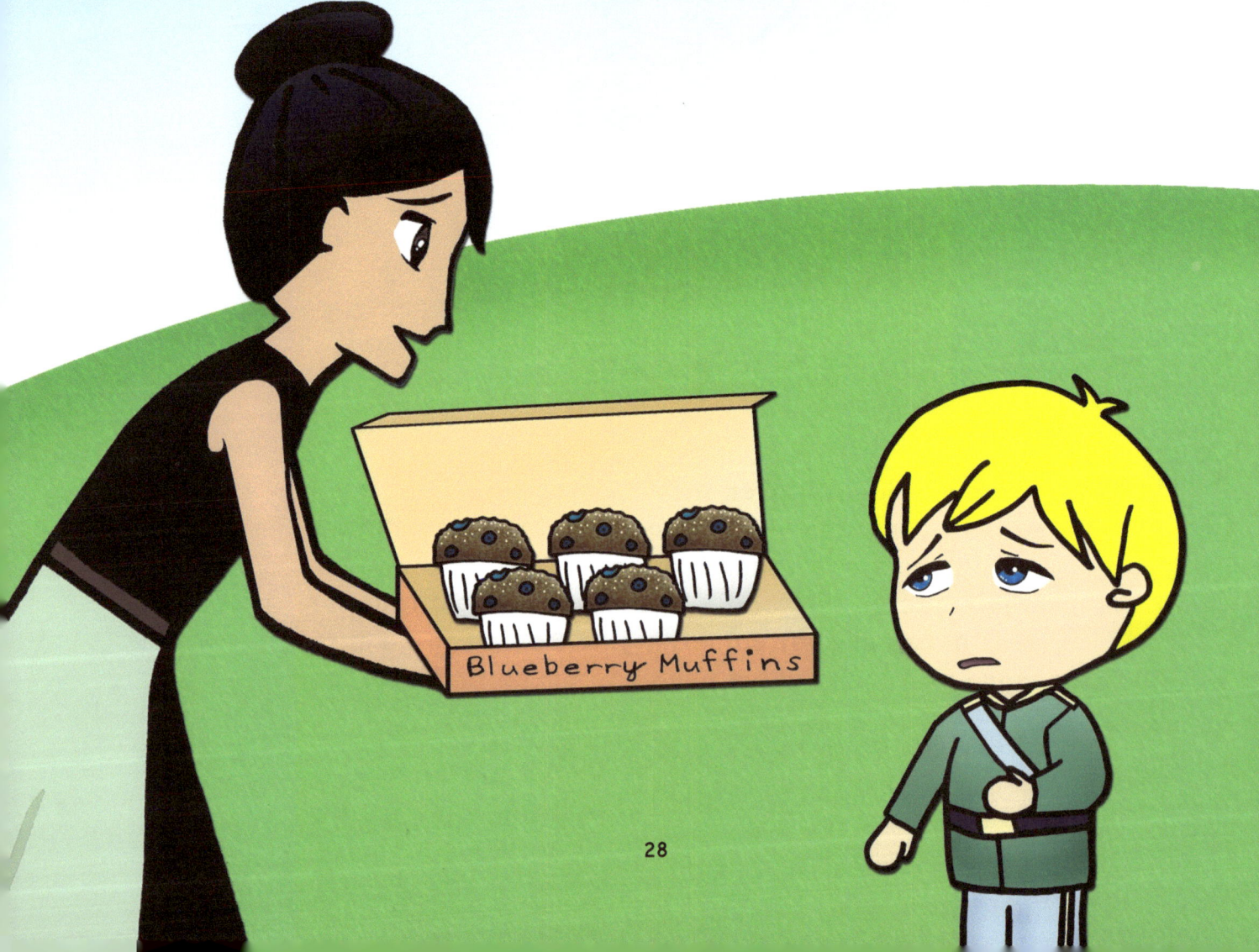

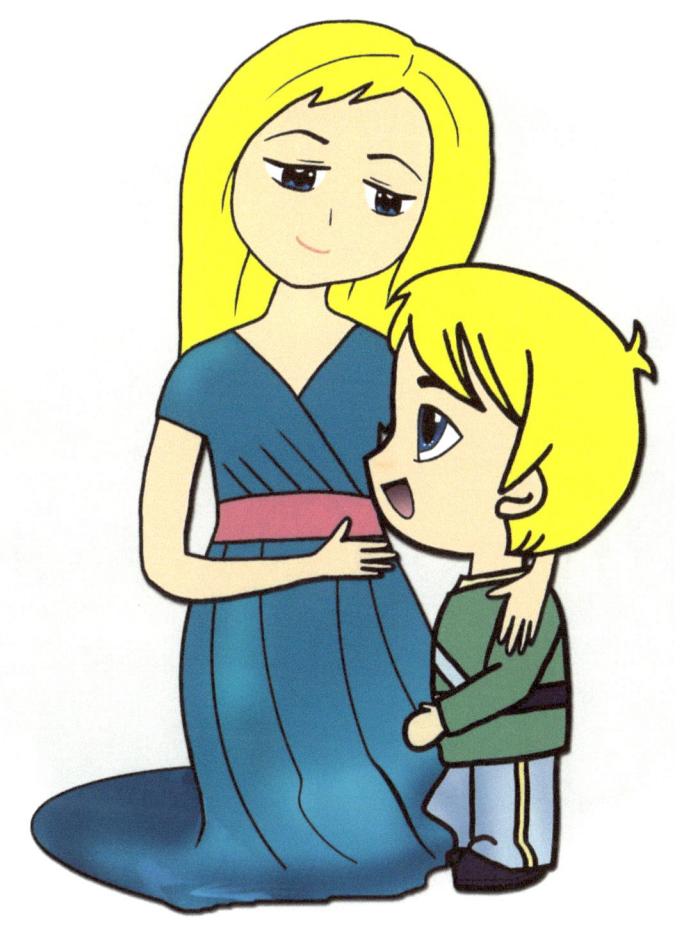

Ethan's mommy put her arm around him.

"I'm proud of you for telling our new friends about your food allergy. Friends care and help keep you safe," she said.

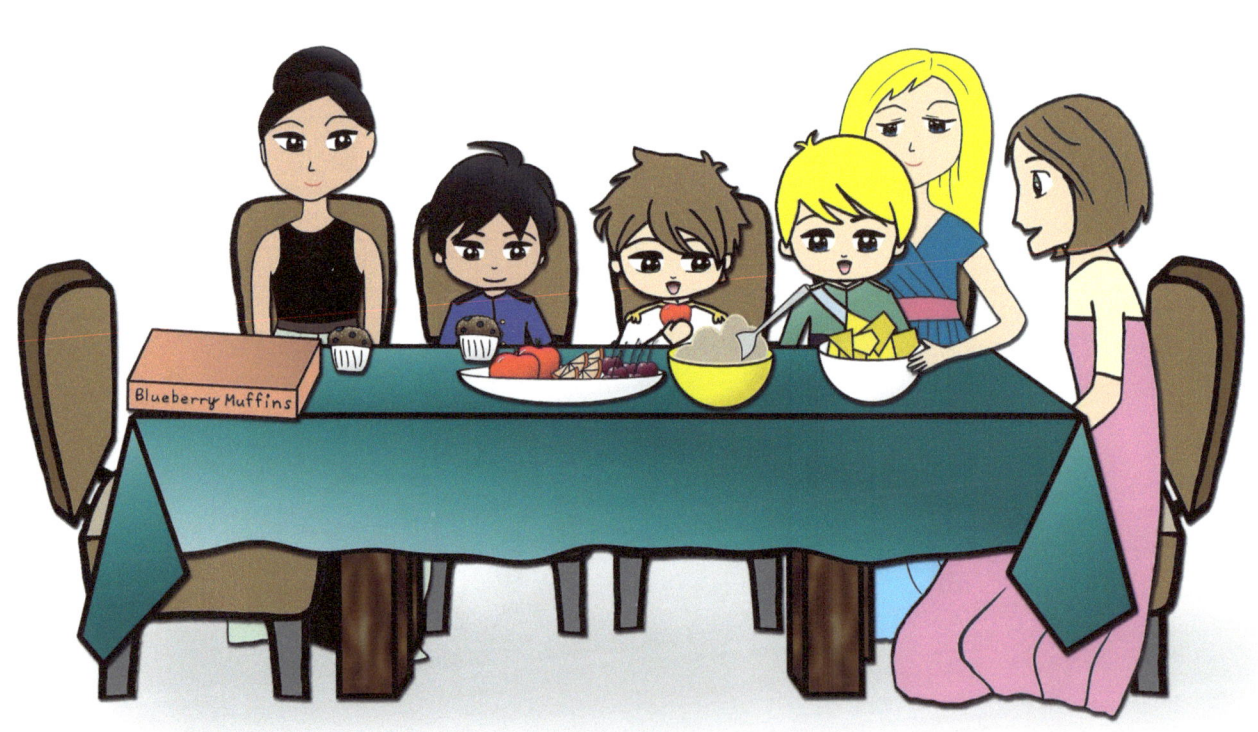

At the table, Ethan reached for the

_____.
[fill in safe snacks here]

"Thank you Mommy for preparing something safe I can eat," said Ethan.

With a loving squeeze, his mommy replied, "I'm always here to keep you safe."

THE END

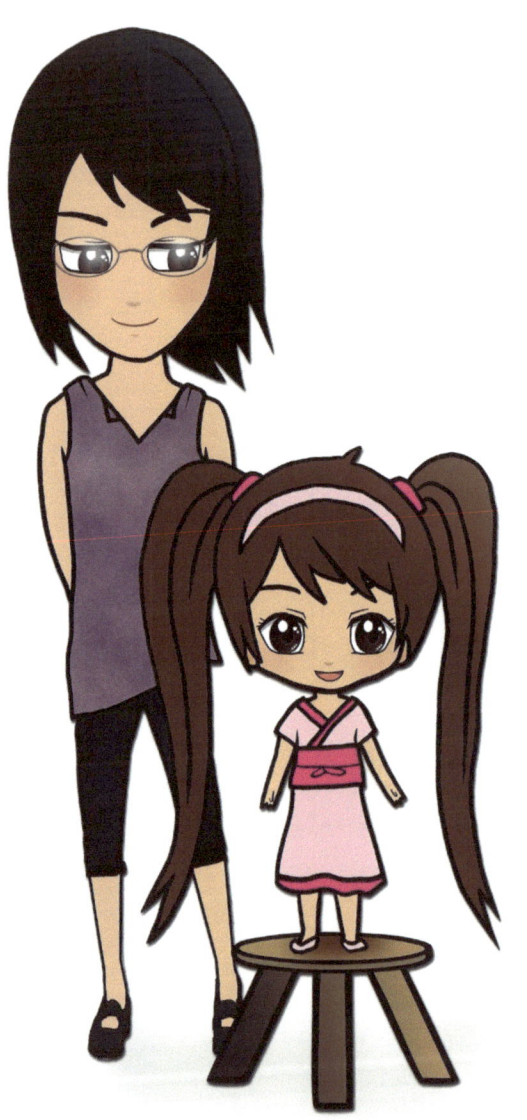

About the Authors

Jennifer Chung was motivated to create this book when she could not find one that targeted her two children's specific food allergies. Despite a love of art, she majored in Computer Science. She remembers receiving strange looks while walking into programming classes with her oversized drawing pad and pastel-smeared jeans. Working on this book with Keira has been the best mother-daughter project ever!

Keira Chung is 11 years old and lives in the USA. She loves gymnastics, violin, and art.

www.AllergicPrince.com

Food Allergy Books

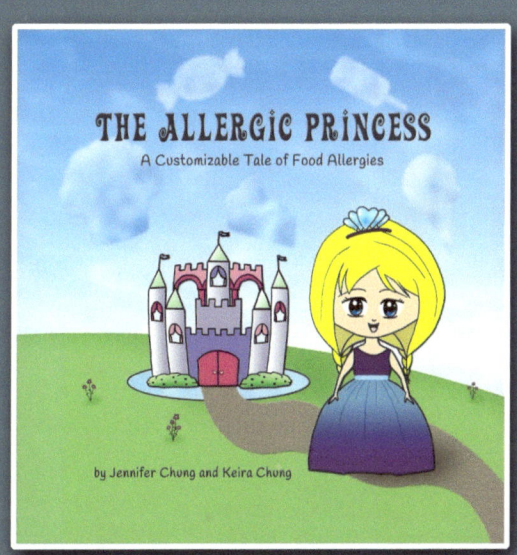

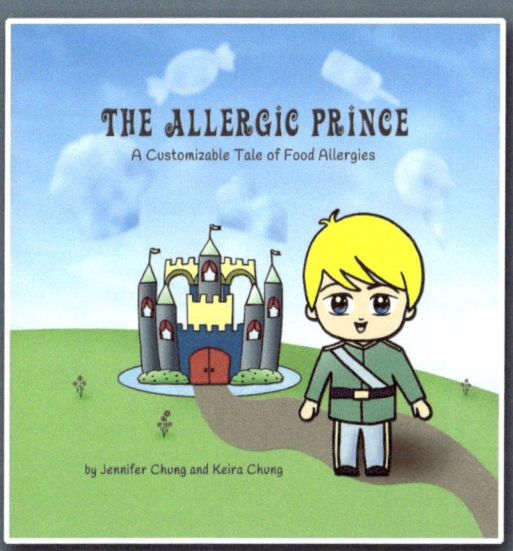

www.AllergicPrincess.com
www.AllergicPrince.com